Guide to Hair Coloring Products

By YANG MUMU

Top 10 Professional Hair Color Brands In The World

Here are the top 10 professional hair color brands in the world, known for their quality and popularity among professional hairstylists:

1. L'Oréal Professionnel: L'Oréal Professionnel is a renowned brand offering a wide range of hair color products, from permanent to semi-permanent and temporary colors. They are known for their innovative formulas and extensive color selection.

2. Wella Professionals: Wella Professionals is a well-established brand with a long history in the hair industry. They offer a wide range of hair color products, including permanent, demi-permanent, and semi-permanent dyes. Wella is known for its high-quality formulas and reliable color results.

3. Redken: Redken is a professional hair care brand that is highly respected in the industry. They offer a variety of hair color options, including vibrant fashion shades and natural-looking tones. Redken's products are known for their long-lasting color and conditioning properties.

4. Schwarzkopf Professional: Schwarzkopf Professional is a popular choice among professional hairstylists. They provide a comprehensive range of hair color products, including permanent, semi-permanent, and lightening options. Schwarzkopf is known for its advanced color technology and extensive shade range.

5. Goldwell: Goldwell is a professional hair color brand that offers vibrant and long-lasting color results. They are known for their high-performance products and innovative color technology. Goldwell

offers a wide range of shades and color lines to cater to different client preferences.

6. Matrix: Matrix is a well-known professional hair care brand that offers a diverse range of hair color products. They provide a variety of color options, from permanent and demi-permanent dyes to balayage and highlighting systems. Matrix is recognized for its color accuracy and versatility.

7. Joico: Joico is a popular brand among professional hairstylists, known for its high-quality hair color products. They offer a wide range of shades and color lines, including vibrant fashion colors. Joico's products are known for their color intensity and long-lasting results.

8. Keune: Keune is a professional hair color brand that combines innovation with quality. They offer a comprehensive range of color options, including permanent, semi-permanent, and ammonia-free dyes. Keune's products are known for their excellent coverage and color longevity.

9. Pravana: Pravana is a brand that is highly regarded for its vibrant and creative hair colors. They specialize in fashion shades and unique color formulations. Pravana's products are known for their bold and vivid color results.

10. Oway: Oway (Organic Way) is a professional hair color brand that focuses on organic and natural ingredients. They offer a range of ammonia-free and vegan hair color options. Oway's products are known for their gentle formulations and eco-friendly approach.

These brands are widely recognized and respected for their quality, innovation, and range of hair color options. It's important to note that individual experiences and preferences may vary, so it's recommended to consult with a professional hairstylist to determine the best hair color brand for your specific needs.

Factors To Consider When Choosing A Permanent Hair Color

When choosing a permanent hair color, there are several factors to consider to ensure you make the right choice. Here are some key factors to keep in mind:

1. Desired Color Result: Think about the specific color result you want to achieve. Consider whether you want a subtle change or a dramatic transformation. Determine if you want to go lighter, darker, or stay within a similar shade range to your natural color. Look for a hair color that offers the shade you desire.

2. Skin Tone: Consider your skin tone when selecting a hair color. Certain shades can complement or clash with your skin tone. Cool-toned skin (with pink or blue undertones) often suits cooler hair colors like ash blondes or cool browns. Warm-toned skin (with yellow or peach undertones) tends to be flattered by warmer hair colors like golden blondes or warm browns. Choosing a color that harmonizes with your skin tone can help create a more flattering overall look.

3. Eye Color: Take into account your eye color as it can be enhanced or complemented by certain hair colors. For example, warm hair colors like copper or golden tones can bring out blue or green eyes, while rich reds or auburns can accentuate brown eyes. Consider how different hair colors might interact with your eye color to create a pleasing effect.

4. Maintenance Level: Permanent hair color is long-lasting and typically requires less frequent touch-ups compared to semi-permanent or temporary options. However, it's essential to consider the maintenance level you're comfortable with. If you prefer low maintenance, choose a color that blends well with your natural hair growth, or opt for shades that fade gracefully without leaving obvious root lines.

5. Hair Condition and Damage: Assess the condition of your hair before selecting a permanent hair color. If your hair is damaged or excessively processed, it may be more vulnerable to further damage from certain hair color formulas. In such cases, choosing a hair color that is gentle and nourishing, or opting for professional salon treatments, might be a better option.

6. Coverage and Gray Hair: If you have gray hair and desire full coverage, make sure to choose a hair color specifically designed to cover grays effectively. Some hair colors have better gray coverage than others, so look for products that specifically mention gray coverage or are formulated for resistant grays if needed.

7. Brand and Product Reputation: Consider the reputation and reliability of the hair color brand and product you are considering. Look for brands with positive reviews, strong customer satisfaction, and a good track record of delivering consistent and high-quality results.

8. Professional Advice: If you're uncertain about which hair color to choose or have specific concerns about your hair, it's always a good idea to consult with a professional hairstylist or colorist. They can provide personalized advice based on their expertise and help you select the best hair color for your individual needs.

By considering these factors, you can make an informed decision and choose a permanent hair color that aligns with your desired outcome and suits your unique features.

67 Types Of Hair Coloring Products

There are numerous types of hair coloring products available in the market. While it is difficult to list all 67 types, here are some common categories of hair coloring products:

1. Permanent hair color

2. Semi-permanent hair color

3. Demi-permanent hair color

4. Temporary hair color

5. Root touch-up products

6. Hair color sprays

7. Hair color mousses

8. Hair color gels

9. Hair color creams

10. Hair color powders

11. Henna hair dye

12. Herbal hair dyes

13. Natural hair colorants

14. Organic hair color

15. Ammonia-free hair color

16. Peroxide-free hair color

17. Bleach powder

18. Developer/activator

19. Toners

20. Color-enhancing shampoos

21. Color-depositing conditioners

22. Color-removing products

23. Color-protecting hair care products

24. Professional salon hair color

25. DIY hair color kits

26. Highlighting kits

27. Balayage kits

28. Ombre kits

29. Color correcting products

30. Gray hair coverage products

31. Fashion/vibrant hair colors

32. Pastel hair colors

33. Metallic hair colors

34. Fantasy hair colors

35. Temporary root touch-up sprays

36. Color refreshers

37. Color-depositing masks

38. Color-boosting serums

39. Color-reviving glosses

40. Root blending powders

41. Tinted dry shampoos

42. Sun-activated hair color

43. Heat-activated hair color

44. Hair color pencils

45. Hair color markers

46. Hair mascara

47. Hair color waxes

48. Hair color remover

49. Color-correcting pens

50. Color-protecting hair serums

51. Color-boosting hair serums

52. Intense color concentrates

53. Pre-color treatments

54. After-color treatments

55. Hair color primers

56. Color-safe hair masks

57. Color-safe hair oils

58. Color-safe hair sprays

59. Color-safe styling products

60. Color-safe heat protectants

61. Temporary color sprays for hair accessories

62. Root concealing powders

63. Hair color touch-up sticks

64. Hair color touch-up pens

65. Gradient hair color products

66. Two-tone hair dye kits

67. Customizable hair color systems

Remember to always follow the instructions and perform patch tests before using any hair coloring product to ensure safety and desired results.

Specific Hair Color Formulas That Are Gentle And Nourishing

I can provide you with some commonly recognized hair color brands known for their gentle and nourishing formulas. It's important to note that formulations and product availability may vary, so it's always a good idea to check for updated information and reviews. Here are a few brands that have been well-regarded for their gentle and nourishing hair color formulas:

1. Olaplex: Olaplex is known for its innovative hair care technology that helps to repair and strengthen damaged hair. They offer a range of hair color products that aim to minimize damage during the coloring process while providing vibrant and long-lasting results.

2. Wella Professionals Koleston Perfect Me+: Wella Professionals Koleston Perfect Me+ is a hair color line that boasts a gentle formula while delivering vibrant and true-to-tone color. It uses a conditioning technology called ME+ that reduces the risk of developing new allergies to hair color.

3. Madison Reed: Madison Reed is a brand that focuses on creating hair color formulations without harsh chemicals like ammonia, resorcinol, and parabens. They offer a wide range of shades and their formulas are enriched with nourishing ingredients like argan oil, keratin, and ginseng root extract.

4. NATURIGIN: NATURIGIN is a brand that specializes in organic and natural hair colors. Their formulations are free from ammonia, resorcinol, and parabens, and instead use certified organic ingredients. They aim to provide a gentle and nourishing coloring experience.

5. dpHUE: dpHUE offers a variety of hair color options, including their Gloss+ line, which is a semi-permanent hair color and deep conditioning treatment in one. Their formulas are free from ammonia, peroxide, and parabens and are designed to add shine, enhance color, and nourish the hair.

Remember to read product labels, descriptions, and customer reviews to ensure that the specific product and shade you choose align with your preferences and needs. Consulting with a professional hairstylist or colorist can also provide valuable insights and recommendations based on your hair's specific condition and requirements.

Hair Color Formulas That Are Gentle And Nourishing For Damaged Hair

Yes, there are hair color formulas available that are specifically formulated to be gentle and nourishing for damaged hair. These formulas often include ingredients that help condition and protect the hair during the coloring process. Here are a few types of hair color formulas known for their gentle and nourishing properties:

1. Ammonia-Free Hair Color: Traditional hair color formulas often contain ammonia, which can be harsh on the hair. Ammonia-free hair

color alternatives use alternative alkaline agents to open the hair cuticle and deposit color. These formulas are generally considered gentler and less damaging to the hair.

2. Oil-Based Hair Color: Some hair color products incorporate oils, such as argan oil, coconut oil, or avocado oil, into their formulas. These oils help to nourish and moisturize the hair, providing added shine and softness. They can also help protect the hair from potential damage caused by the coloring process.

3. Conditioning Hair Color: Certain hair color formulas include conditioning agents that help hydrate and repair the hair while coloring. These formulas often contain ingredients such as proteins, vitamins, or botanical extracts that aim to improve the hair's condition and provide extra moisture.

4. Gentle or Low-Ammonia Hair Color: Some hair color brands offer gentle or low-ammonia hair color options. These products contain reduced amounts of ammonia compared to traditional formulas, which can help minimize potential damage to the hair while still providing long-lasting color results.

5. Demi-Permanent Hair Color: Demi-permanent hair color is a less damaging alternative to permanent hair color. It doesn't contain ammonia and uses a lower volume developer, which is less harsh on the hair. Demi-permanent color typically fades gradually over time and doesn't provide full gray coverage, but it can be a good option for those with damaged hair seeking a more gentle coloring process.

When choosing a hair color specifically for damaged hair, look for products that explicitly mention their gentle or nourishing properties. Read product labels, descriptions, and customer reviews to ensure that the formula aligns with your specific needs. It's also beneficial to consult with a professional hairstylist or colorist who can recommend hair color options that are best suited to your hair's condition and needs.

The Best + Worst Box Hair Color

Best: Professional salon-grade box hair color with high-quality ingredients and a wide range of shades.

Worst: Cheap box hair color with harsh chemicals, limited color options, and poor color payoff.

The best and worst box hair color can vary depending on personal preference, hair type, and desired results. However, here are some general considerations:

Best Box Hair Color:

1. L'Oréal Paris Excellence Crème: Known for its rich and long-lasting color, this brand offers a wide range of shades and provides good gray coverage.

2. Clairol Natural Instincts: This semi-permanent hair color is ammonia-free and provides a natural-looking result with subtle dimension.

3. Garnier Nutrisse: This brand offers a variety of shades and is enriched with nourishing ingredients like avocado oil, shea butter, and olive oil.

4. Revlon Colorsilk: It is an affordable option that delivers vibrant color and provides decent gray coverage.

5. Schwarzkopf Keratin Color: This brand is known for its conditioning properties and vibrant color results.

Worst Box Hair Color:

1. Generic or unknown brands: It's generally recommended to avoid unknown or generic brands as they may have lower-quality ingredients and result in poor color payoff and uneven application.

2. Overly cheap or discounted products: Extremely inexpensive hair color products may contain harsh chemicals that can damage your hair or result in unpredictable color results.

3. Products with high ammonia content: Hair color with high ammonia content can cause strong chemical smells and potential damage to your hair.

4. Poorly reviewed products: Before purchasing a box hair color, check reviews and ratings from other users to get an idea of the product's performance and potential issues.

It's important to keep in mind that box hair color may not always produce the same results as professional salon color. If you have specific concerns or want a major hair color change, it's recommended to consult a professional hairstylist for personalized advice and assistance.

Some Specific Ingredients Or Features To Look For When Choosing A Box Hair Color

When choosing a box hair color, there are specific ingredients and features you can look for to help ensure a more favorable experience and result. Here are some key factors to consider:

1. Ammonia-Free or Low Ammonia: Ammonia is a common ingredient in hair color that helps open the hair cuticle for color penetration. However, it can be harsh and cause damage to the hair. Look for ammonia-free or low ammonia formulas, which can be gentler and less damaging to the hair.

2. Conditioning and Nourishing Ingredients: Hair color can be drying to the hair, so opt for formulas that contain conditioning and nourishing ingredients. Examples include natural oils (such as avocado oil, olive oil, or argan oil), shea butter, aloe vera, or proteins

like keratin. These ingredients can help nourish and moisturize the hair during the coloring process.

3. Color-Protecting Ingredients: Some box hair color brands include ingredients that help protect and preserve the color, such as UV filters or antioxidants. These ingredients can help prevent color fading and extend the vibrancy of your hair color.

4. Gray Hair Coverage: If you have gray hair and want to achieve full coverage, look for box hair color specifically formulated to cover gray hair effectively. These colors often have stronger pigments or specialized formulations to ensure better coverage on resistant gray strands.

5. Application Tools and Accessories: Consider the tools and accessories included in the box hair color kit. Look for applicator bottles or brushes that make the application process easier and more precise. Gloves, conditioning treatments, or post-coloring care products included in the kit can also be beneficial.

6. Color Chart and Shade Selection: Check if the brand provides a color chart or shade swatches to help you choose the right color for your desired result. Having a variety of shades to choose from can increase the likelihood of finding a color that matches your preference.

7. Patch Test and Safety Precautions: Ensure that the box hair color includes instructions for conducting a patch test to check for potential allergic reactions. Safety precautions and detailed instructions for proper application should also be provided in the package.

Remember, while box hair color can be convenient, it may not provide the same level of customization and expertise as a professional salon service. If you have specific concerns or desired results, consulting with a professional hairstylist is recommended.

Box Dye Vs Professional Colour

Box dye and professional color both have their pros and cons. Here are some factors to consider when comparing box dye and professional color:

Box Dye:

- Convenience: Box dye is readily available at drugstores and can be used at home, providing a convenient option for those who prefer to dye their hair on their own schedule.

- Affordability: Box dye is generally more affordable compared to professional color services at a salon.

- Limited customization: Box dye offers a range of pre-mixed shades, but the options for customization and achieving complex color results may be limited.

- Potential risks: Box dye may contain harsh chemicals that can damage hair if not used properly. It's important to follow the instructions carefully and perform a patch test to avoid adverse reactions.

Professional Color:

- Expertise and customization: Professional colorists have the knowledge and expertise to create customized color formulations and achieve complex color results. They can assess your hair type, condition, and desired outcome to create a personalized color plan.

- Higher quality products: Professional color products typically contain higher-quality ingredients, which can result in better color payoff, longevity, and less damage to the hair.

- Skillful application: Professional colorists have the training and experience to apply color evenly and precisely, ensuring optimal results.

- Additional services: Salons often offer additional services like color correction, highlights, and balayage techniques that may not be achievable with box dye.

Ultimately, the choice between box dye and professional color depends on your preferences, desired results, and budget. If you're looking for a simple color refresh or subtle change, box dye can be a convenient and affordable option. However, for more complex color transformations or if you have specific hair concerns, consulting a professional colorist is recommended to achieve the best results while minimizing potential risks.

Real Hairdresser Puts The Best Box Hair Dye To The Test…Shocking Results

When a real hairdresser puts "the best" box hair dye to the test and claims to have "shocking results," it suggests that they have evaluated the performance of a specific box hair dye brand or product and were surprised by the outcome. The phrase "the best" implies that the hairdresser has chosen a highly regarded or recommended box hair dye brand for their test.

The hairdresser's evaluation may include factors such as color accuracy, ease of application, coverage of gray hair, longevity of the color, and overall satisfaction with the results. By referring to the results as "shocking," the hairdresser likely means that they were pleasantly surprised or impressed by the quality or performance of the box hair dye, possibly exceeding their initial expectations.

It's important to remember that the effectiveness of box hair dye can vary depending on individual factors such as hair type, condition, and starting color, as well as the specific brand and shade used. Results can also be influenced by the hairdresser's expertise and technique in applying the dye.

While the hairdresser's review may be informative and valuable, it's essential to consider that their experience represents their personal opinion and may not be universally applicable. Different individuals may have different preferences, hair types, and desired outcomes when it comes to hair dye.

If you're considering using a box hair dye based on a hairdresser's recommendation or review, it can be helpful to research the brand, read reviews from other users, and consider consulting with a professional stylist or colorist who can provide personalized advice based on your specific hair needs and goals.

Ultimately, the results and satisfaction with box hair dye will vary from person to person, and it's important to carefully follow the instructions provided with the product and perform any necessary patch or strand tests before applying the dye to your entire head of hair.

I Put Box Dye To The Test

Putting box dye to the test typically refers to experimenting with or evaluating the performance and results of a commercially available hair dye kit that can be purchased in a box.

When putting box dye to the test, individuals often assess various aspects such as color accuracy, ease of application, coverage of gray hair, longevity of the color, and overall satisfaction with the results. They may compare the box dye to professional salon dye or other hair coloring methods to determine its effectiveness and value.

It's important to note that the results of using box dye can vary depending on factors such as the individual's hair type, condition, and starting color, as well as the specific brand and shade of box dye used. Some people may have successful experiences with box dye, achieving their desired color and satisfactory results, while others may encounter challenges or less-than-desirable outcomes.

When conducting a box dye test, it's recommended to carefully follow the instructions provided with the specific kit, perform a patch test to check for any allergic reactions or sensitivities, and consider doing a strand test to preview the color outcome before applying it to the entire head.

Additionally, it's important to be aware of the limitations of box dye compared to professional salon services. Box dyes typically provide a more limited range of color options, may not be able to achieve drastic color changes or lightening, and may not offer the same level of customization and expertise as a professional colorist.

If you're considering using box dye, it can be helpful to research different brands, read reviews from other users, and consult with a hairstylist for recommendations or advice based on your specific hair type and desired outcome.

Overall, putting box dye to the test involves evaluating the performance, results, and overall satisfaction of using a commercially available hair dye kit. It can provide insights into the effectiveness and suitability of box dye for individual hair coloring needs but keep in mind that the results can vary.

How To Dye Your Hair At Home Like A Pro With Sally's Products

Dyeing your hair at home can be a fun and cost-effective way to change your look. Sally Beauty is a popular retailer that offers a wide range of hair dye products. Here's a step-by-step guide on how to dye your hair at home like a pro using Sally's products:

1. Choose the right hair dye: Sally Beauty carries a variety of hair dye brands, so select one that suits your needs. Consider factors like the color you want to achieve, whether you want permanent or semi-permanent color, and any special considerations for your hair type.

2. Gather your supplies: Apart from the hair dye, you'll need a few additional supplies. These typically include gloves, an applicator brush or bottle, a mixing bowl, an old towel or cape, a hair clip or elastic, and petroleum jelly or barrier cream to protect your skin.

3. Do a patch test: Before applying the hair dye all over your head, it's essential to perform a patch test to check for any allergic reactions. Follow the instructions provided with the hair dye for the patch test procedure.

4. Prepare your work area: Set up a clean and well-lit area for dyeing your hair. Cover surfaces with newspapers or plastic sheets to protect them from any potential stains.

5. Protect your clothing: Wear an old shirt or drape a towel around your shoulders to shield your clothing from the hair dye.

6. Section your hair: Divide your hair into manageable sections using clips or elastics. This will make it easier to apply the dye evenly and ensure complete coverage.

7. Follow the instructions: Carefully read the instructions provided with the hair dye. The instructions will vary depending on the brand and type of dye you're using. Pay attention to recommended development times, application techniques, and any additional steps specific to the product.

8. Mix the dye: If your hair dye requires mixing, follow the instructions provided to prepare the dye mixture. This may involve combining colorant and developer in a specific ratio. Use the mixing bowl and applicator brush provided or use your own clean tools if necessary.

9. Apply the dye: Start applying the hair dye to your hair, working one section at a time. Use the applicator brush or bottle to distribute the dye evenly from roots to ends. Ensure that each strand is thoroughly coated with dye.

10. Time the process: Set a timer according to the instructions to ensure that you leave the dye on for the recommended duration. This is crucial for achieving the desired color and preventing over-processing.

11. Rinse and condition: Once the development time is complete, rinse your hair thoroughly with lukewarm water until the water runs clear. Follow up with a conditioner to help restore moisture to your hair. Some hair dye kits may include a conditioner specifically designed for use after coloring.

12. Style and assess the results: After rinsing and conditioning, style your hair as desired. Take a look at the final result to see if it matches your expectations. If you're satisfied, great! If not, you may need to make adjustments or consult a professional stylist for further assistance.

Remember, dyeing your hair at home carries some risks, especially if you're inexperienced or trying a drastic color change. If you're unsure or have concerns about the process, it's always a good idea to consult a professional hair colorist.

Recommend Some Specific Sally's Hair Dye Products That Are Beginner-Friendly

Here are a few beginner-friendly hair dye products from Sally Beauty that you can consider:

1. Ion Color Brilliance Permanent Creme Hair Color: Ion is a popular brand known for its wide range of hair color options. Their Color Brilliance line offers permanent hair dye in various shades. The formula is easy to use and provides long-lasting results.

2. Arctic Fox Semi-Permanent Hair Color: Arctic Fox is a vegan and cruelty-free brand that offers a range of vibrant semi-permanent hair colors. These dyes are easy to apply and do not require any

developer or mixing. They are also gentle on the hair and can be mixed to create custom shades.

3. Clairol Professional Soy4Plex LiquiColor Permanente: Clairol is a trusted brand in the hair dye industry. Their Soy4Plex LiquiColor Permanente provides long-lasting color and 100% gray coverage. The formula contains soy protein to nourish and protect the hair during the coloring process.

4. Wella Color Charm Permanent Liquid Hair Color: Wella Color Charm is a reliable brand that offers a range of permanent hair dyes. The liquid formula is easy to mix and apply, making it suitable for beginners. They offer a wide selection of shades, including natural tones and vibrant colors.

5. L'Oreal Excellence Creme Permanent Hair Color: L'Oreal is a well-known brand in the beauty industry, and their Excellence Creme line offers a range of permanent hair colors. The formula is easy to use and provides full coverage and long-lasting results. It also includes a conditioning treatment to help nourish the hair after coloring.

Remember to carefully read the instructions and choose a shade that is close to your natural hair color or within a few shades of it for the best results, especially if you're a beginner. Additionally, performing a strand test before applying the dye all over your hair is always recommended to preview the color outcome and check for any adverse reactions.

Hair Dye Products That Are Specifically Recommended For Sensitive Scalps

There are hair dye products available that are specifically formulated for individuals with sensitive scalps. These products often have milder formulas and ingredients that are less likely to cause irritation. Here are a few options to consider:

1. Naturtint Permanent Hair Color: Naturtint is a brand that offers permanent hair color products that are free from ammonia, parabens, and other harsh chemicals. They use plant-based ingredients and botanical extracts to provide gentle and nourishing color. Naturtint is known for being suitable for sensitive scalps and for those with allergies.

2. Herbatint Permanent Hair Color Gel: Herbatint is a gentle, ammonia-free hair color gel that is formulated with natural ingredients. It is free from harsh chemicals and has a low allergy risk. The formula is designed to be gentle on the scalp while providing long-lasting color.

3. Madison Reed Radiant Hair Color Kit: Madison Reed offers a range of hair color kits that are formulated without ammonia, parabens, resorcinol, and other potentially irritating ingredients. Their products are designed to be gentle and nourishing to the hair and scalp. Madison Reed also provides an online color matching service to help you find the right shade.

4. Surya Brasil Henna Cream: Surya Brasil offers a henna-based hair coloring cream that is free from ammonia, peroxide, and other harsh chemicals. Henna is a natural alternative that can be gentler on the scalp. The cream is enriched with plant extracts and moisturizing ingredients to provide a conditioning effect.

5. Tints of Nature Permanent Hair Color: Tints of Nature is a brand that focuses on using natural and organic ingredients in their hair color products. Their formulas are free from ammonia, parabens, and resorcinol. They are known for being gentle on the scalp and for providing vibrant, long-lasting color.

When choosing a hair dye for sensitive scalps, it's always a good idea to perform a patch test before applying the dye all over your head. This can help you determine if you have any adverse reactions to the product. Additionally, it's a good practice to follow the instructions provided with the hair dye and to consult with a dermatologist or allergist if you have specific concerns about your scalp's sensitivity.

Natural Or Organic Hair Coloring Products Available In The Market

Yes, there are natural and organic hair coloring products available in the market. These products are often formulated with plant-based ingredients and exclude synthetic chemicals such as ammonia, parabens, and sulfates. They aim to provide a more natural and gentle alternative to traditional hair dyes. Here are a few examples of natural and organic hair coloring options:

1. Henna: Henna is a plant-based hair dye that has been used for centuries. It is often considered a natural and safe alternative to chemical hair dyes. Henna imparts a reddish-brown color to the hair and can also provide conditioning benefits.

2. Plant-Based Hair Dyes: Some companies offer hair dyes made from plant-based ingredients such as herbal extracts, fruits, and flowers. These dyes often come in powder or liquid form and provide a range of natural shades. They are typically free from harsh chemicals and are intended to be gentle on the hair and scalp.

3. Organic Hair Color Brands: Several brands specialize in organic and natural hair color products. They use certified organic ingredients and avoid synthetic chemicals. These brands often offer a wide range of shades and products, including permanent, semi-permanent, and temporary hair dyes.

4. Henna-Based Creams: Some brands offer henna-based hair coloring creams that combine henna with other natural ingredients. These creams are designed to provide a wider range of color options and can be a more convenient alternative to traditional henna powders.

5. Botanical Hair Color: Botanical hair color products use a combination of natural botanical extracts and pigments to achieve color results. They are formulated without ammonia, peroxide, and synthetic dyes. Botanical hair color products are often marketed as a gentle and natural option.

It's important to note that even natural and organic hair coloring products may cause allergic reactions or sensitivities in some individuals. It's advisable to perform a patch test and carefully read and follow the instructions provided by the manufacturer. Additionally, the color results and longevity of natural and organic hair dyes may vary compared to traditional dyes, so it's important to set realistic expectations.

Benefits Of Using Natural And Organic Hair Coloring Products Compared To Traditional Dyes

Using natural and organic hair coloring products can offer several benefits compared to traditional dyes that contain synthetic chemicals. Here are some advantages:

1. Reduced Chemical Exposure: Natural and organic hair coloring products often exclude harsh chemicals like ammonia, parabens, and sulfates. By choosing natural alternatives, you can minimize your exposure to potentially harmful substances that may be found in traditional hair dyes.

2. Gentler on the Hair and Scalp: Natural and organic hair coloring products tend to be milder and gentler on the hair and scalp. They often contain nourishing ingredients that can help condition and moisturize the hair, reducing the likelihood of damage and dryness.

3. Less Risk of Allergic Reactions: Synthetic chemicals in traditional hair dyes can cause allergic reactions in some individuals. Natural and organic hair coloring products, especially those formulated with

plant-based ingredients, are generally considered to have a lower risk of causing allergic sensitivities.

4. Environmentally Friendly: Many natural and organic hair coloring products are produced using sustainable and eco-friendly practices. They often use plant-based ingredients that are renewable and biodegradable, reducing the environmental impact compared to traditional dyes.

5. Potential Health Benefits: Some natural ingredients used in organic hair coloring products, such as henna, may offer additional health benefits. For example, henna has been traditionally used to promote scalp health, strengthen hair, and add natural shine.

6. Variety of Shades: Natural and organic hair coloring products come in a variety of shades, allowing you to achieve different color results while still opting for a more natural approach. These products often provide more subtle tones and earthy hues that blend well with natural hair colors.

It's important to note that natural and organic hair coloring products may have some limitations compared to traditional dyes. They may have different color results, may not provide as much color longevity, or may not be able to lighten the hair as dramatically. It's recommended to carefully read the instructions and choose a product that aligns with your desired outcome and hair type.

Specific Natural Ingredients That Are Commonly Used In Organic Hair Coloring Products

Organic hair coloring products often incorporate a variety of natural ingredients to achieve color and provide nourishment to the hair. Here are some commonly used natural ingredients in organic hair coloring products:

1. Henna (Lawsonia inermis): Henna is a plant-based dye that has been used for centuries to color hair. It provides a reddish-brown color and is known for its conditioning properties. Henna can help strengthen the hair, add shine, and improve overall hair health.

2. Indigo (Indigofera tinctoria): Indigo is another natural plant-based dye commonly used in organic hair coloring products. It produces shades of blue or black when combined with henna. Indigo is often used in combination with henna to achieve a wider range of colors, including brown and black.

3. Cassia (Cassia obovata): Cassia, also known as neutral henna, is a plant that provides a yellowish-golden color when used as a hair dye. It can be used alone or in combination with other natural dyes to achieve different shades.

4. Chamomile (Matricaria chamomilla): Chamomile is often used in hair care products, including organic hair coloring products, due to its lightening and brightening properties. It can help add golden or blonde highlights to the hair naturally.

5. Beetroot (Beta vulgaris): Beetroot extract is sometimes used as a natural dye to add a reddish or purplish tint to hair. It can be found in certain organic hair coloring products, especially those that offer vibrant or unconventional shades.

6. Amla (Emblica officinalis): Amla, also known as Indian gooseberry, is a common ingredient in Ayurvedic hair care. It is rich in vitamin C and antioxidants and is believed to promote hair growth and strengthen the hair. Amla is sometimes used in organic hair coloring products to provide conditioning benefits.

7. Coffee (Coffea arabica): Coffee can be used as a natural dye to add a temporary brown tint to the hair. It is often used in homemade hair rinses or as an ingredient in organic hair color products to achieve subtle brown shades.

These are just a few examples of natural ingredients commonly used in organic hair coloring products. Each brand may have its own unique blend of natural ingredients to create their formulations. It's important to read the product labels or consult with the manufacturer to determine the specific ingredients in a particular organic hair coloring product.

Fast & Easy Time-saving Hair Coloring Tips & Techniques

Here are some fast and easy time-saving hair coloring tips and techniques:

1. Prep Your Hair: Before starting the coloring process, make sure your hair is clean and free of any styling products. This will help the color adhere better to your hair.

2. Choose a Single-Process Color: If you're short on time, opt for a single-process color instead of complex techniques like highlights or ombre. Single-process color involves applying a single shade all over your hair, which is quicker and easier to do.

3. Use a Hair Color Kit: Hair color kits come with all the necessary tools and instructions for at-home coloring. They are designed to be user-friendly and time-saving. Follow the instructions carefully to achieve the desired results.

4. Focus on the Roots: Instead of coloring your entire hair from roots to ends every time, focus on coloring just the regrowth or roots. This will save time and reduce damage to the lengths of your hair.

5. Section Your Hair: Divide your hair into sections using clips or hair ties before applying the color. This will help you apply the color evenly and efficiently.

6. Quick Application Techniques: If you're pressed for time, consider using quick application techniques like the "squeeze bottle" or "comb and drag" methods. These techniques allow you to apply color to small sections of hair more quickly.

7. Opt for Express Color Products: Some hair color products are designed for quick processing times. Look for express color formulas that can develop in a shorter amount of time, saving you precious minutes.

8. Consider Dry Shampoo Color: Dry shampoo color products are a convenient option for touch-ups and temporary color. They can quickly refresh your hair color without the need for washing and drying.

9. Protect Your Skin: Apply a thin layer of petroleum jelly or a barrier cream around your hairline, ears, and neck to prevent staining from the hair color. This will make cleanup easier and faster.

10. Follow Proper Aftercare: After coloring your hair, follow the recommended aftercare instructions to maintain the color and keep your hair healthy. This includes using color-safe shampoos and conditioners and minimizing heat styling.

Remember, if you're unsure or have specific hair color concerns, it's always best to consult a professional hairstylist. They can provide personalized advice and ensure you achieve the desired results.

Recommended Brands Or Products For Quick-Processing Hair Color

There are several brands that offer quick-processing hair color products designed to reduce the development time and provide faster results. Here are a few recommended options:

1. L'Oréal Excellence Creme: L'Oréal Excellence Creme is a popular hair color brand that offers a variety of shades and also includes a quick-processing formula called "Excellence Quick." This line is specifically formulated to provide full coverage and vibrant color in a shorter processing time.

2. Clairol Natural Instincts: Clairol Natural Instincts is known for its semi-permanent hair color options that offer a quick development time. The color typically develops in about 10 minutes, making it a convenient choice for those looking for a faster coloring process.

3. Garnier Nutrisse Express Retouch: Garnier Nutrisse Express Retouch is a root touch-up product that is designed to cover gray roots in just 10 minutes. It comes in a convenient pen-like format with a precision applicator, allowing for targeted and quick application.

4. Revlon Colorsilk Beautiful Color: Revlon Colorsilk Beautiful Color is a widely available and affordable hair color brand. While it doesn't have a specific quick-processing line, many users have reported that the color develops relatively quickly compared to other brands, often within 25-30 minutes.

5. Schwarzkopf Simply Color: Schwarzkopf Simply Color is a hair color brand that offers a quicker processing time compared to traditional color formulas. It is free from ammonia, silicone, and alcohol, and provides coverage and vibrancy in about 30 minutes.

It's important to note that the processing time can vary depending on factors such as the desired color result, hair type, and the specific product you're using. Always refer to the instructions provided with the product for accurate processing times and guidelines.

Additionally, it's recommended to perform a patch test and conduct a strand test before using any hair color product to ensure compatibility and to preview the color result. If you have specific hair concerns or are unsure about the best product for your needs, it's advisable to consult with a professional hairstylist or colorist for personalized recommendations.

Hair Color Products That Provide Faster Results

Certainly! Here are a few hair color products known for providing faster results:

1. Schwarzkopf Keratin Color: Schwarzkopf Keratin Color is a hair color line that offers vibrant and long-lasting results. It is formulated with keratin to help improve hair strength and has a development time of approximately 30 minutes, which is relatively shorter compared to some other brands.

2. Clairol Nice 'n Easy Perfect 10: Clairol Nice 'n Easy Perfect 10 is designed to provide full coverage and vibrant color in just 10 minutes. It is a permanent hair color option that offers quick results and is available in a range of shades.

3. Garnier Olia: Garnier Olia is an ammonia-free hair color line that is known for its vibrant and rich color results. It utilizes an oil-based formula that helps to nourish and hydrate the hair. The processing time for Garnier Olia is typically around 30 minutes.

4. L'Oréal Paris Feria: L'Oréal Paris Feria is a hair color line that offers a wide range of bold and vibrant shades. It provides intense color results and typically has a processing time of approximately 25-30 minutes.

5. Revlon ColorSilk: Revlon ColorSilk is a budget-friendly hair color option that is widely available. While the processing time can vary depending on the specific shade and product, many ColorSilk formulations develop in approximately 25-30 minutes.

Remember to carefully read and follow the instructions provided with the product you choose, as processing times can vary depending on factors such as the desired color result and hair type. Additionally, it's advisable to perform a patch test and conduct a strand test prior to full application to ensure compatibility and preview the color outcome.

If you have specific hair concerns or are looking for personalized recommendations, it's always a good idea to consult with a professional hairstylist or colorist.

How To Color Your Hair And Beard

Coloring your hair and beard can be done using similar techniques. Here's a general guide on how to color your hair and beard:

1. Choose the Right Color: Select a hair color and beard color dye that matches or complements your desired shade. Consider factors such as your skin tone, natural hair color, and personal preference.

2. Gather the Supplies: Get all the necessary supplies, including hair dye for your hair, beard dye specifically formulated for facial hair, gloves, mixing bowl, applicator brush, plastic or disposable cape, petroleum jelly or barrier cream, and a timer.

3. Perform a Patch Test: Before applying the dye to your hair or beard, it's important to perform a patch test to check for any allergic reactions. Apply a small amount of the dye mixture behind your ear or on the inner side of your wrist and leave it for the recommended time. If you experience any discomfort or irritation, do not proceed with coloring.

4. Prepare the Dye: Follow the instructions provided with the hair dye and beard dye to prepare the mixture. Usually, this involves mixing the hair dye and developer in the provided mixing bowl.

5. Protect Your Skin: Apply a thin layer of petroleum jelly or a barrier cream around your hairline, ears, and neck to protect your skin from staining.

6. Apply the Hair Dye: Start by applying the hair dye to your hair. Section your hair using clips or hair ties and use an applicator brush to apply the dye evenly to each section. Make sure to saturate the hair strands from roots to ends. Follow the recommended processing time mentioned in the instructions.

7. Apply the Beard Dye: After applying the hair dye, move on to the beard. Use an applicator brush or the provided brush to apply the beard dye to your facial hair. Start from the areas with the most gray or desired color change, and work your way through the rest of the beard. Make sure to cover the beard evenly and thoroughly. Follow the recommended processing time.

8. Rinse and Shampoo: Once the processing time is complete, rinse both your hair and beard thoroughly with lukewarm water until the water runs clear. Follow up with a color-safe shampoo to remove any remaining dye residue. Condition your hair and beard as usual.

9. Style as Desired: After coloring, style your hair and beard as desired. You can use styling products, such as pomade or beard oil, to achieve the desired look and maintain the color.

It's important to read and follow the instructions provided with the hair dye and beard dye carefully. If you're unsure or have specific concerns, it's recommended to consult a professional hairstylist or barber for guidance. They can provide personalized advice and ensure you achieve the best results while minimizing the risk of damage or color mishaps.

Common Mistakes To Avoid When Coloring Your Hair And Beard At Home

When coloring your hair and beard at home, it's important to be mindful of certain common mistakes to avoid. Here are some key ones:

1. Skipping the Patch Test: Always perform a patch test before applying the hair dye or beard color to your entire hair or beard. This helps identify any potential allergic reactions or adverse effects. Follow the instructions provided with the product for conducting a patch test.

2. Not Reading the Instructions: Carefully read and follow the instructions provided with the hair dye or beard color product. Each product may have specific guidelines regarding mixing ratios, application techniques, and processing times. Skipping or misinterpreting the instructions can lead to undesired results.

3. Neglecting Strand Testing: Conduct a strand test before applying the color to your entire hair or beard. This involves applying the dye to a small section of hair to assess the color outcome and processing time. It helps ensure that you achieve the desired shade and also determine the appropriate processing time.

4. Applying the Color Unevenly: Take care to apply the hair dye or beard color evenly to ensure uniform color results. Section your hair or beard and use an applicator brush or comb to distribute the color thoroughly from roots to ends. Uneven application can result in splotchy or patchy color.

5. Choosing the Wrong Color Shade: Selecting the wrong color shade is a common mistake. Consider factors such as your natural hair color, skin tone, and personal preference when choosing a shade. If unsure, it's advisable to consult with a professional hairstylist or colorist for guidance.

6. Overlapping Color on Previously Colored Hair: If you're retouching or coloring over previously colored hair, avoid overlapping the color onto the already colored sections. Overlapping can lead to excessive color buildup, uneven color, or damage to the hair.

7. Leaving the Color on for Too Long: Adhering to the recommended processing time is crucial. Leaving the color on for longer than

instructed can lead to over-processing, hair damage, or undesired color results. Set a timer to ensure you follow the specified processing time.

8. Failing to Maintain and Care for Colored Hair: Colored hair requires proper maintenance and care to preserve the color and keep the hair healthy. Use color-safe shampoos and conditioners, avoid excessive heat styling, and protect your hair from sun exposure to prevent color fading.

If you're uncertain about any step of the process or have specific concerns, it's always advisable to seek guidance from a professional hairstylist or colorist. They can provide personalized advice and help you achieve the best results.

Tips For Choosing The Right Hair Dye Or Beard Color Shade

Choosing the right hair dye or beard color shade is crucial to achieving a desired and flattering result. Here are some tips to help you select the appropriate shade:

1. Consider Your Natural Hair Color: Take your natural hair color into account when choosing a shade. If you want a subtle change or minimal maintenance, opt for a color that is close to your natural shade. If you're looking for a more dramatic transformation, you can choose a shade that is significantly lighter or darker than your natural color.

2. Determine Your Skin Tone: Your skin tone plays a role in determining which hair dye or beard color shade will suit you best. Generally, cool-toned skin (with pink or blue undertones) is complemented by cool hair colors like ash blondes, cool browns, or blacks. Warm-toned skin (with yellow or peach undertones) tends to be flattered by warm hair colors like golden blondes, copper reds, or warm browns.

3. Assess Your Eye Color: Consider your eye color when selecting a hair dye or beard color shade. Certain colors can enhance or complement your eye color. For example, warm hair colors like golden or honey tones can bring out blue or green eyes, while rich reds or auburns can accentuate brown eyes.

4. Determine Your Desired Intensity: Decide on the level of intensity you want for your hair or beard color. Are you looking for a subtle change or a bold transformation? If you're unsure, you can start with a semi-permanent or temporary dye to test out a shade before committing to a permanent color.

5. Seek Professional Advice: If you're uncertain about which shade would suit you best, consider consulting with a professional hairstylist or colorist. They can assess your hair, skin tone, and features to provide personalized recommendations based on their expertise.

6. Use Online Tools and Apps: Some hair dye brands and online platforms offer virtual hair color try-on tools or apps. These tools allow you to upload a photo and virtually try out different hair colors and shades to visualize how they might look on you. While not always 100% accurate, they can give you a general idea of how a particular shade might suit you.

Remember that hair dye and beard color can appear slightly different on different individuals due to variations in natural hair color, texture, and porosity. It's always a good idea to perform a strand test before applying the color to your entire hair or beard to ensure you achieve the desired outcome.

Ultimately, choosing a hair dye or beard color shade is a personal decision, so go with the shade that makes you feel confident and reflects your individual style.

Do Wish Hair Color Products Work On Dark Hair

Wish is an online marketplace that offers a wide range of products, including hair color products. However, since Wish is a platform where multiple sellers list their products, it's crucial to note that the quality and effectiveness of hair color products can vary significantly. It's always recommended to carefully read product descriptions, customer reviews, and consider the reputation of the seller before making a purchase.

In general, when it comes to coloring dark hair, achieving vibrant or light shades can be more challenging compared to coloring lighter hair. Dark hair often contains more pigment, which can require additional steps or specialized products to achieve desired results. Some hair color products may specifically mention their suitability for dark hair or offer formulas designed to work on darker shades.

To effectively color dark hair, it may be necessary to lighten or pre-lighten the hair before applying a desired color. This process can involve using bleach or other lightening agents to lift the hair's natural pigment and create a base for the desired hair color to show up more vividly.

It's important to note that the outcome will also depend on factors such as the specific product used, the starting color of your hair, the health and condition of your hair, and the application technique. For more complex or drastic color changes, it's generally recommended to consult with a professional hairstylist or colorist who can provide personalized advice and assistance.

Before using any hair color product, particularly on dark hair, it's advisable to perform a strand test to assess how the color will appear and to check for any adverse reactions. Additionally, following the product's instructions carefully and taking proper aftercare measures can help maintain the color and overall health of your hair.

Specific Techniques Or Tips For Coloring Dark Hair With Hair Color Products

Coloring dark hair with hair color products can require specific techniques and considerations to achieve desired results. Here are some techniques and tips to keep in mind when coloring dark hair:

1. Pre-Lightening: If you want to achieve vibrant or light shades on dark hair, pre-lightening or bleaching may be necessary. This process involves using a bleach or lightening product to lift the natural pigment in the hair, creating a lighter base for the desired color. It's important to follow the instructions carefully and perform a strand test to assess the level of lightening required and ensure the hair's integrity.

2. Developer Strength: When using permanent hair color, the developer or peroxide strength plays a crucial role in lightening dark hair. Higher volume developers, such as 30 or 40, can lift more pigment but may also cause more damage. It's generally recommended to start with a lower volume developer and gradually increase if needed, especially if you're coloring your hair at home.

3. Choose the Right Hair Color: Select a hair color shade that is specifically formulated for dark hair or offers vibrant results on darker shades. Look for shades specifically designed for dark hair or those that are labeled as "high lift" or "intense" colors. These shades often contain more pigment and are formulated to provide better coverage and vibrancy on dark hair.

4. Sectioning and Application: Divide your hair into sections and apply the hair color product evenly from roots to ends. Dark hair can be more resistant to color, so make sure to saturate the hair thoroughly and evenly to ensure consistent results. It can be helpful to use clips or hair ties to keep sections separate and work methodically from one section to another.

5. Processing Time: Follow the recommended processing time specified by the hair color product. Dark hair may require longer processing times to achieve desired results. However, it's important to avoid leaving the color on for longer than recommended, as it can lead to damage or an undesired outcome.

6. Maintenance and Aftercare: After coloring your dark hair, it's important to follow proper aftercare to maintain the color and the health of your hair. Use color-safe shampoos and conditioners formulated for color-treated hair, avoid excessive heat styling, and protect your hair from prolonged sun exposure. Regular touch-ups may also be necessary to maintain the vibrancy of the color.

Keep in mind that achieving drastic color changes, especially on dark hair, can be challenging and may require professional assistance. If you're unsure or seeking more complex color transformations, consulting with a professional hairstylist or colorist is recommended to ensure the best possible outcome while minimizing potential damage.

Tips For Maintaining The Color And Vibrancy Of Dark Hair After Coloring

Certainly! Here are some tips for maintaining the color and vibrancy of dark hair after coloring:

1. Use Color-Safe Hair Care Products: Opt for shampoos, conditioners, and styling products specifically formulated for color-treated hair. These products are designed to be gentle and help preserve the color by minimizing fading. Look for sulfate-free formulas, as sulfates can strip away color.

2. Wash Hair Less Frequently: Washing your hair less often can help preserve the color. Try to extend the time between washes and use dry shampoo or other hair-refreshing products to keep your hair looking clean and fresh between washes. When you do wash your

hair, use lukewarm water instead of hot water, as hot water can cause color to fade faster.

3. Cold Rinse: After shampooing and conditioning, finish your shower with a cold water rinse. Cold water helps seal the hair cuticle, locking in the color and adding shine. It may be a bit uncomfortable, but it can make a difference in preserving your color.

4. Protect from UV Exposure: Prolonged sun exposure can cause color fading, especially for dark hair. Protect your hair from UV rays by wearing a hat or using hair products with UV protection when you're going to be exposed to the sun for an extended period.

5. Minimize Heat Styling: Heat styling tools like flat irons, curling irons, and blow dryers can contribute to color fading. Minimize the use of these tools or use them on lower heat settings. Apply a heat protectant spray before styling to create a barrier between your hair and the heat.

6. Deep Conditioning Treatments: Regular deep conditioning treatments help keep your hair moisturized and nourished, which can enhance the vibrancy of the color. Look for deep conditioning masks or treatments specifically formulated for color-treated hair and use them as recommended.

7. Avoid Chlorine and Saltwater: Chlorine in pools and saltwater can strip away color and cause it to fade more quickly. If you plan to swim, wet your hair with clean water before entering the pool or ocean to minimize absorption. You can also use a leave-in conditioner or hair oil to create a barrier between your hair and the water.

8. Regular Touch-Ups: Depending on the rate of hair growth and the desired level of color vibrancy, regular touch-ups may be necessary. Consult with a professional colorist to determine the ideal frequency for touch-ups based on your specific hair and color needs.

By following these tips, you can help maintain the color and vibrancy of your dark hair for longer periods between coloring sessions. Remember that each hair is unique, so it's a good idea to consult with a professional hairstylist or colorist who can provide personalized advice based on your hair type and color-treated hair needs.

Natural Remedies Or Diy Treatments That Can Help Maintain The Color Of Dark Hair

While natural remedies and DIY treatments may not be as potent as professional hair care products, they can still provide some beneficial effects for maintaining the color of dark hair. Here are a few natural remedies and DIY treatments you can try:

1. Vinegar Rinse: Rinse your hair with a mixture of apple cider vinegar and water after shampooing and conditioning. The acidity of vinegar helps to seal the hair cuticle, enhance shine, and preserve the color. Mix one part vinegar with three parts water and pour it over your hair as a final rinse. Rinse thoroughly afterward to remove the vinegar scent.

2. Black Tea Rinse: Brew strong black tea and let it cool down. After shampooing, pour the black tea over your hair as a final rinse. Black tea contains tannins that can help darken and enrich the color of dark hair. Leave the tea on for a few minutes before rinsing it out with cool water.

3. Coffee Rinse: Brew a strong pot of coffee, allow it to cool, and then use it as a hair rinse after shampooing. Coffee can help enhance the depth of dark hair color. Pour the cooled coffee over your hair, leave it on for a few minutes, and then rinse it out thoroughly.

4. Henna Treatment: Henna is a natural plant-based dye that can be used to enhance and maintain dark hair color. Look for high-quality,

pure henna powder without any additives or chemicals. Follow the instructions on the henna package to create a paste, apply it to your hair, and leave it on for the recommended time before rinsing it out. Henna can provide a reddish tint to dark hair and also acts as a natural conditioner.

5. Aloe Vera Gel: Aloe vera gel is known for its moisturizing and nourishing properties. Apply fresh aloe vera gel or store-bought pure aloe vera gel to your hair and scalp. Leave it on for about 30 minutes before rinsing it out. Aloe vera can help keep your hair hydrated and healthy, which can contribute to maintaining the color.

6. Coconut Oil Treatment: Coconut oil is a popular natural hair treatment that can help strengthen and moisturize the hair. Apply warm coconut oil to your hair, focusing on the ends and dry areas. Leave it on for at least 30 minutes or overnight before shampooing it out. Regular coconut oil treatments can help maintain the overall health and shine of your hair, which can enhance the appearance of the color.

Remember that natural remedies and DIY treatments may have subtle effects and may not provide the same long-lasting results as professional hair care products. It's essential to be patient and consistent when using these treatments and to understand that individual results may vary. If you have any concerns or questions, it's always recommended to consult with a professional hairstylist or colorist.

5 Best Permanent Hair Colors To Buy In 2024

I can give you a list of popular permanent hair color brands that have been well-regarded in the past. Keep in mind that preferences and availability can vary, so it's always a good idea to research and read reviews before making a purchase. Here are five reputable permanent hair color brands that have been popular:

1. L'Oréal Paris Excellence Creme: L'Oréal Paris is known for its wide range of hair color products, and Excellence Creme is a popular choice for permanent hair color. It offers a variety of shades and provides long-lasting color with gray coverage.

2. Garnier Nutrisse: Garnier Nutrisse is another well-known brand that offers a range of permanent hair color options. Their formula is enriched with nourishing ingredients and provides vibrant color results.

3. Clairol Nice'n Easy: Clairol Nice'n Easy has been a trusted brand for permanent hair color for many years. They offer a wide selection of shades, including natural-looking colors and multi-dimensional tones.

4. Schwarzkopf Keratin Color: Schwarzkopf is a reputable brand in the hair care industry, and their Keratin Color line offers permanent hair color with intense and long-lasting results. The formula is designed to improve the hair's structure and shine.

5. Wella Professionals Koleston Perfect: Wella Professionals is a widely recognized brand among hairstylists and salon professionals. Their Koleston Perfect line offers vibrant and true-to-tone permanent hair color with a wide range of shades.

Remember to carefully follow the instructions provided with the hair color product and conduct a patch test before applying it to your entire hair to check for any allergic reactions or sensitivities.

It's always a good idea to consult with a professional hairstylist for personalized advice and to choose the best permanent hair color specifically suited to your hair type, desired results, and any specific concerns you may have.

Coloring My Hair Twice With Simpler Hair Color

Coloring your hair twice with a simpler hair color can be done, but there are a few things to consider to achieve desired results while maintaining hair health:

1. Wait for a sufficient interval: It's important to allow an appropriate amount of time between hair coloring sessions to minimize damage and prevent over-processing. Waiting at least 4-6 weeks between colorings is generally recommended.

2. Choose a gentle hair color: Opt for a hair color that is ammonia-free and contains conditioning ingredients to minimize damage and maintain the health of your hair. Look for products labeled as "gentle" or "nourishing" to ensure a milder formulation.

3. Consider the color change: If you're planning to change your hair color significantly with the second application, it's important to assess the compatibility of the new color with your current hair color. For example, going from a dark shade to a lighter color may require pre-lightening or bleaching your hair to achieve the desired result.

4. Protect and nourish your hair: Using hair care products specifically designed for color-treated hair can help maintain the vibrancy and health of your hair. Use sulfate-free shampoos and conditioners formulated for color-treated hair, and consider using hair masks or deep conditioners regularly to nourish and hydrate your strands.

5. Seek professional advice if unsure: If you're uncertain about the hair coloring process or want to achieve a specific result, it's always a good idea to consult a professional hairstylist. They can assess your hair condition, provide guidance on color selection and application techniques, and help you achieve your desired outcome while minimizing potential damage.

Remember, repeated hair coloring can affect the condition of your hair, so it's essential to prioritize hair health and take proper care of your locks throughout the process.

The Hair Color That Will Best Suit Your Skin Tone

Choosing a hair color that complements your skin tone can enhance your overall appearance. While individual preferences and personal style play a role in hair color selection, here are some general guidelines to consider:

1. Warm Skin Tone:

   - Best Hair Colors: Warm tones like golden blonde, honey blonde, caramel, copper, and auburn can complement warm skin tones. Rich browns with warm undertones, such as chestnut or chocolate, can also be flattering.

   - Avoid: Cool tones like platinum blonde or ash brown may clash with warm skin tones.

2. Cool Skin Tone:

   - Best Hair Colors: Cool tones like platinum blonde, ash blonde, ash brown, cool chocolate, and burgundy can complement cool skin tones. Jewel-toned hair colors like sapphire blue or emerald green can also be striking.

   - Avoid: Warm tones with reddish or golden undertones may not harmonize with cool skin tones.

3. Neutral Skin Tone:

   - Best Hair Colors: Neutral skin tones have the flexibility to pull off a wide range of hair colors. You can experiment with both warm and cool tones to find what suits your personal style. Natural shades like medium brown, dark blonde, or soft black often work well.

   - Avoid: There are no strict color restrictions for neutral skin tones, so feel free to explore different options.

It's important to keep in mind that these are general guidelines, and personal preferences and style should ultimately dictate your hair color choice. Additionally, consider factors such as eye color, natural hair color, and lifestyle when selecting a hair color that reflects your personality and enhances your overall look.

If you're uncertain about which hair color will suit you best, consulting with a professional hairstylist can provide valuable insights and personalized recommendations based on your specific features and preferences.

What's the Difference Between Permanent, Demi & Semi-Permanent Hair Colors

The main differences between permanent, demi-permanent, and semi-permanent hair colors lie in their formulation, application process, and longevity:

1. Permanent Hair Color:

   - Formulation: Permanent hair color contains ammonia and oxidative agents, such as hydrogen peroxide, which permanently alter the hair's natural pigment.

   - Coverage and Color Change: Permanent color can provide full coverage for gray hair and can create significant color changes, such as lightening dark hair or going from lighter to darker shades.

   - Longevity: Permanent color lasts until it grows out or is cut off. The new hair growth at the roots will be your natural color, and touch-ups are needed to maintain the desired shade.

2. Demi-Permanent Hair Color:

   - Formulation: Demi-permanent hair color is ammonia-free and uses a lower concentration of oxidative agents compared to permanent color. It deposits color onto the hair shaft without significantly lightening the natural pigment.

   - Coverage and Color Change: Demi-permanent color can provide excellent coverage for gray hair, but it is generally used to enhance or deepen the current hair color rather than for drastic color changes.

   - Longevity: Demi-permanent color typically lasts through 20-28 shampoos. It gradually fades over time but does not leave a clear demarcation line as the hair grows out.

3. Semi-Permanent Hair Color:

   - Formulation: Semi-permanent hair color is free of ammonia and oxidative agents. It coats the hair shaft with color rather than penetrating it.

   - Coverage and Color Change: Semi-permanent color is mainly used to enhance the natural hair color, add subtle highlights, or experiment with temporary fashion shades. It cannot lighten the hair or provide full coverage for gray hair.

   - Longevity: Semi-permanent color lasts through 4-12 shampoos, gradually fading with each wash. It does not leave a demarcation line as the hair grows out.

When choosing between permanent, demi-permanent, and semi-permanent hair color, consider your desired level of permanence, the extent of color change you want to achieve, and the amount of maintenance you're willing to commit to. It's also important to follow the instructions provided with the specific hair color product for the best results and to maintain the health of your hair.

Specific Hair Care Practices That Can Help Prolong The Longevity Of Demi-Permanent Or Semi-Permanent Hair Color

There are several hair care practices that can help prolong the longevity of demi-permanent or semi-permanent hair color. While these types of color will eventually fade over time, proper care can help extend their vibrancy and keep the color looking fresh. Here are some tips:

1. Wait before shampooing: After coloring your hair with demi-permanent or semi-permanent color, wait at least 24 to 48 hours before shampooing. This allows the color molecules to fully settle into the hair shaft and helps improve color retention.

2. Use color-safe and sulfate-free products: Regular shampoos can strip the color from your hair, so opt for color-safe shampoos and conditioners specifically formulated for colored hair. Look for products that are sulfate-free, as sulfates can be harsh and cause color fading. These products are designed to be gentler on the hair and help preserve the color.

3. Wash with cool water: Hot water can open the hair cuticles and cause color molecules to escape more quickly. When rinsing your hair, use cool or lukewarm water to help seal the cuticles and keep the color intact.

4. Limit washing frequency: Washing your hair too frequently can lead to color fading. Try to extend the time between washes to allow the color to last longer. Use dry shampoo or other styling products to refresh your hair between washes if needed.

5. Minimize heat styling: Heat styling tools like flat irons, curling irons, and blow dryers can cause color to fade more quickly. Limit the use of heat styling tools or use them on lower heat settings to minimize damage and color loss. Consider using heat protectant sprays before using any heat styling tools.

6. Protect your hair from the sun: UV rays can fade hair color, so protect your hair from excessive sun exposure. Wear a hat, use UV-

protective hair products, or apply a leave-in conditioner with UV filters before going out in the sun.

7. Deep condition regularly: Demi-permanent and semi-permanent colors can sometimes make the hair slightly more porous, so it's important to keep the hair moisturized and nourished. Use deep conditioning treatments or hair masks regularly to help maintain the health of your hair and prolong the color's vibrancy.

8. Avoid chlorine and saltwater: Chlorine in swimming pools and saltwater can be harsh on colored hair and cause color fading. Before swimming, wet your hair with clean water and apply a leave-in conditioner or hair oil to create a protective barrier. After swimming, rinse your hair thoroughly to remove any chlorine or saltwater.

By following these hair care practices, you can help prolong the longevity of your demi-permanent or semi-permanent hair color and keep your hair looking vibrant and fresh for a longer period.

My Favorite Hair Color Lines And Why I Use So Many Different Brands! Permanent, Demi, Direct Dyes

I can provide you with information about popular hair color lines that are favored by many individuals. Here are some well-known hair color brands that offer a range of permanent, demi-permanent, and direct dye options:

1. L'Oréal Paris: L'Oréal Paris is a widely recognized brand known for its extensive range of hair color products. They offer permanent hair color lines like Excellence Creme and Preference, as well as demi-permanent options like Casting Creme Gloss. L'Oréal also offers direct dye options like Colorista, which allows for temporary and vibrant color transformations.

2. Wella Professionals: Wella Professionals is a professional hair care brand that provides a variety of hair color options. Their permanent hair color line, Koleston Perfect, offers a wide range of shades and provides long-lasting results. For demi-permanent color, Wella offers Color Touch, which offers shine and conditioning benefits. They also have direct dye options like Color Fresh Create for vibrant temporary colors.

3. Schwarzkopf Professional: Schwarzkopf Professional is known for its high-quality hair color products. Their permanent hair color line, Igora Royal, offers a vast range of shades and provides excellent coverage and color retention. Schwarzkopf also offers demi-permanent color options like Igora Vibrance, which provides intense shine and lasts up to 25 washes. They have direct dye options like Igora Colorworx for creative color applications.

4. Joico: Joico is a popular brand among hairstylists and enthusiasts for their innovative hair color lines. Their permanent hair color line, Joico Color Intensity, offers vibrant and long-lasting colors. Joico also offers demi-permanent color options like LumiShine, which provides nourishing and conditioning benefits. For direct dyes, Joico Color Intensity Eraser allows for easy color removal and correction.

5. Pravana: Pravana is well-known for its vivid and creative color options. Their permanent hair color line, Pravana ChromaSilk, offers vibrant and long-lasting colors in a wide range of shades. Pravana also provides a semi-permanent color line called Pravana Vivids, which offers bold and vibrant direct dye options for temporary color transformations.

These are just a few examples of popular hair color brands that offer permanent, demi-permanent, and direct dye options. Each brand may have its own unique features, such as color range, longevity, conditioning properties, or creative possibilities. It's common for individuals to use different brands based on their specific color preferences, desired effects, and experiences with different products. Experimenting with different brands allows for versatility and the ability to achieve diverse color results.

Specific Uv-Protective Hair Products To Use For Sun Protection

Here are a few specific UV-protective hair products that you can consider:

1. Sun Bum 3-In-1 Leave-In Hair Conditioning Treatment: Sun Bum offers a 3-in-1 leave-in conditioning treatment that provides UV protection for the hair. It helps to protect against sun damage, minimize color fading, and nourish the hair with key ingredients like coconut oil and banana peel extract.

2. Aveda Sun Care Protective Hair Veil: Aveda Sun Care Protective Hair Veil is a lightweight mist that provides UV defense for the hair. It helps to protect against the harmful effects of the sun, minimize color fading, and prevent dryness and damage. It also contains antioxidants to help protect the hair from environmental stressors.

3. Biolage Sunsorials Sunflower Color Preserving Hair Oil: Biolage Sunsorials Sunflower Color Preserving Hair Oil is formulated to protect color-treated hair from the sun's harmful rays. It contains sunflower seed oil, which helps to prevent color fading and provides UV protection. It also helps to add shine and control frizz.

4. Paul Mitchell Sun Shield Conditioning Spray: Paul Mitchell Sun Shield Conditioning Spray is a leave-in conditioner that provides UV protection for the hair. It helps to shield the hair from sun damage, prevent color fading, and keep the hair moisturized and healthy. It also detangles the hair and adds shine.

5. Redken Color Extend Sun Take Cover Protective Spray: Redken Color Extend Sun Take Cover Protective Spray is specifically designed to protect color-treated hair from UV rays. It helps to

prevent color fading, minimize damage, and keep the hair hydrated. It also provides a lightweight, non-greasy finish.

When using UV-protective hair products, make sure to follow the instructions provided by the manufacturer. Apply the product to damp or dry hair before sun exposure, and reapply as necessary throughout the day, especially after swimming or excessive sweating.

Remember that in addition to using UV-protective products, wearing a hat or scarf and limiting direct sun exposure during peak hours can also help protect your hair from the damaging effects of the sun.

Other Ways To Protect Hair From The Sun Besides Using Uv-Protective Products

There are other ways to protect your hair from the sun besides using UV-protective products. Here are some additional measures you can take:

1. Wear a Hat or Scarf: One of the most effective ways to shield your hair from the sun is by wearing a wide-brimmed hat or a scarf. These accessories provide physical protection by creating a barrier between your hair and the sun's rays. Opt for hats or scarves made from tightly woven materials for better sun protection.

2. Limit Sun Exposure: Minimize direct sun exposure during peak hours, typically between 10 a.m. and 4 p.m. If you know you'll be spending an extended period in the sun, try to seek shade or take breaks in shaded areas to reduce the amount of time your hair is exposed to sunlight.

3. Protective Hairstyles: Styling your hair in updos, braids, or other protective hairstyles can help shield your strands from sun exposure. By keeping your hair off your shoulders and away from direct sunlight, you reduce the amount of UV radiation it receives.

4. Rinse with Clean Water: Before swimming in a pool or the ocean, wet your hair with clean water. This helps to minimize the absorption of chlorinated or saltwater, which can have drying and damaging effects on your hair. Rinsing afterward with clean water can also help remove residual chemicals.

5. Avoid Heat Styling: Reduce the use of heat styling tools like blow dryers, curling irons, and flat irons during periods of sun exposure. Heat can further dehydrate your hair, making it more susceptible to damage from the sun's rays. Embrace natural hairstyles or air-dry your hair when possible.

6. Hydrate and Moisturize: Keeping your hair well-hydrated and moisturized can help fortify its natural defenses against sun damage. Use hydrating hair masks, conditioners, and leave-in treatments to nourish your hair and maintain its moisture balance.

7. Regular Trims: Trim your hair regularly to remove split ends and prevent further damage. Trimming helps to maintain the overall health of your hair and can minimize the impact of sun-related damage.

Remember, while these measures can help protect your hair from the sun, they may not provide complete UV protection. Using UV-protective products in combination with these practices will give you the best defense against sun damage.

Examples Of Uv-Protective Products That Can Be Used To Protect Hair From The Sun

There are several UV-protective hair products available in the market that can help protect your hair from the sun's harmful rays. Here are some examples:

1. Leave-In Conditioners with UV Protection: Many leave-in conditioners are formulated with UV filters to shield the hair from sun

damage. Look for products specifically labeled as "UV protection" or "sun protection" leave-in conditioners. These products typically provide hydration, detangling benefits, and UV defense in one.

2. Hair Sprays with UV Filters: Some hair sprays contain UV filters that create a protective barrier on the hair strands. These sprays can be applied before sun exposure to shield the hair from harmful UV rays. Look for hair sprays that mention UV protection or sun protection on the label.

3. UV-Protective Hair Serums: There are hair serums available that are specially formulated with UV protection properties. These serums often contain lightweight, non-greasy formulas that provide a layer of protection and leave the hair smooth and shiny. Apply a small amount of the serum to your hair before heading out in the sun.

4. Hair Oils with UV Filters: Certain hair oils come with added UV filters to protect the hair from sun damage. These oils can be used as a pre-styling treatment or applied to dry hair to provide sun protection and nourishment. Look for hair oils that contain UV filters or mention sun protection on the packaging.

5. UV-Protective Leave-In Sprays: Leave-in sprays specifically designed for sun protection offer an easy and convenient way to shield your hair from the sun. These sprays often have lightweight formulas that can be applied before and during sun exposure to provide continuous UV defense.

It's important to note that the level of UV protection may vary among products, so look for those that offer broad-spectrum protection against both UVA and UVB rays. Additionally, remember to follow the instructions provided by the manufacturer for proper application and reapplication of the products.

Keep in mind that while these products can provide some level of UV protection, they are not a substitute for other sun protection measures such as wearing a hat or seeking shade when the sun's rays are strongest. Combining these products with other sun protection practices will help ensure the best possible protection for your hair.

How To Use Just For Men Original Formula - Shampoo-in Color

To use Just For Men Original Formula - Shampoo-in Color, follow these steps:

1. Start with dry, unwashed hair. Put on the gloves provided in the box to protect your hands.

2. Squeeze out equal amounts of the color base and color developer into the mixing tray. Use the comb provided to mix them together until they are thoroughly blended.

3. Apply the mixture to your dry hair using the comb. Start at the areas where you have the most gray hair and work your way through the rest of your hair.

4. Make sure to completely saturate your hair with the mixture, especially the gray areas. Use the comb to spread the color evenly and ensure thorough coverage.

5. Leave the color on your hair for the recommended amount of time indicated in the instructions. This is usually around 5 minutes.

6. Rinse your hair thoroughly with warm water until the water runs clear. Avoid getting the color on your skin or eyes.

7. Shampoo your hair with a mild shampoo and rinse again. Condition your hair as usual.

8. Style your hair as desired once it is dry.

Remember to carefully read and follow the instructions provided in the Just For Men Original Formula - Shampoo-in Color box for best results.

Can I Use Just For Men Original Formula On My Beard Or Mustache As Well

Yes, Just For Men Original Formula can be used on both your beard and mustache. It is specifically designed to color facial hair and provides natural-looking results.

When using Just For Men Original Formula on your beard or mustache, you can follow a similar application process as you would for your hair:

1. Choose the Right Color: Select the shade of Just For Men Original Formula that matches your natural beard or mustache color or the color you desire.

2. Perform a Patch Test: It's important to conduct a patch test on a small area of your skin to check for any allergic reactions or sensitivity. Follow the patch test instructions provided in the product packaging.

3. Prepare the Area: Protect your clothing and the surrounding area by placing an old towel or cape around your shoulders and covering surfaces that may come into contact with the product.

4. Mix the Color: Open the Just For Men Original Formula package and mix the color base tube and developer as directed in the instructions. Shake the mixture well to ensure thorough mixing.

5. Apply the Color: Wearing gloves (provided in the package), apply the mixed color to your dry beard or mustache. Use your fingers or a small brush to apply the color evenly, making sure to fully saturate the hair.

6. Wait and Rinse: Leave the color on your beard or mustache for the recommended amount of time specified in the instructions. Check the mirror to monitor the color development. Once the desired color is achieved, rinse your beard or mustache thoroughly with warm water until the water runs clear.

7. Apply Color-Protecting Conditioner: After rinsing, apply the color-protecting conditioner provided in the Just For Men Original Formula package. Massage it into your beard or mustache and leave it on for a couple of minutes. Then, rinse it out thoroughly.

8. Style as Desired: Once your beard or mustache is clean and conditioned, you can style it as you normally would.

Always read and follow the instructions provided with the Just For Men Original Formula package when coloring your beard or mustache. If you have any concerns or questions, consult the included instructions or contact the manufacturer's customer service for assistance.

Is Just For Men Original Formula Safe To Use On Sensitive Skin

Just For Men Original Formula is generally well-tolerated by most individuals, including those with sensitive skin. However, it's important to note that everyone's skin is unique, and some individuals may have sensitivities or allergies to certain ingredients.

Before using Just For Men Original Formula or any hair color product on your skin, it's recommended to perform a patch test. Apply a small amount of the product mixture on a small area of skin, such as the inside of your forearm or behind your ear. Leave it on for the recommended time specified in the instructions and then rinse it off. Monitor the test area for any signs of redness, irritation, or allergic reactions, such as itching or swelling, for the next 48 hours. If you experience any adverse reactions, do not use the product.

If you have a history of skin sensitivities or allergies, or if you're uncertain about using Just For Men Original Formula on your sensitive skin, it's advisable to consult a dermatologist or healthcare professional before proceeding. They can evaluate your specific situation and provide personalized guidance.

Additionally, carefully follow the instructions provided with the product and avoid contact with the skin as much as possible during the application process. Applying a thin layer of petroleum jelly or a similar protective barrier around the hairline and skin areas can help minimize potential staining.

Overall, while Just For Men Original Formula is generally safe for use, it's important to be mindful of your individual skin sensitivities and perform a patch test to ensure compatibility before applying it to larger areas or sensitive skin.

How To Color Your Hair: A Better Alternative To Just For Men - Simpler Hair Color Product Review

To color your hair, follow these general steps:

1. Choose the right hair color product: Look for a hair color product that suits your needs and preferences. Consider factors such as the desired color, coverage, and any specific requirements for your hair type.

2. Read the instructions: Before using any hair color product, carefully read the instructions provided by the manufacturer. Pay attention to the recommended application process, development time, and any safety precautions.

3. Do a patch test: Perform a patch test to check for any potential allergic reactions or sensitivity to the hair color product. Apply a small amount of the mixture on a small area of your skin, typically behind the ear or on the inner forearm, and wait for the recommended time.

If you experience any adverse reactions, do not proceed with the hair color application.

4. Prep your hair: Start with clean, dry hair. Remove any styling products, oils, or residue that might interfere with the color application. It's recommended to shampoo your hair the day before coloring and avoid using conditioner or styling products on the day of coloring.

5. Protect your clothing and surroundings: Wear an old shirt or use a hair coloring cape to protect your clothes from any potential stains. Cover surfaces with old towels or plastic sheets to prevent staining your countertops or floors.

6. Mix the hair color: Follow the instructions to mix the hair color product. Typically, you'll need to combine the colorant with the developer in a specific ratio. Use a plastic or glass bowl and a brush or applicator provided with the product to mix them thoroughly.

7. Apply the color: Start applying the hair color from the roots, working your way towards the ends. Use the brush or applicator to ensure even distribution of the color. If you have long or thick hair, section it off for easier application. Avoid applying the color to your scalp to minimize staining.

8. Wait for the development time: Follow the recommended development time indicated in the instructions. This allows the color to process and penetrate the hair shaft. Use a timer to keep track of the time accurately.

9. Rinse and condition: After the development time, rinse your hair thoroughly with lukewarm water until the water runs clear. Apply the conditioner provided with the hair color product or a deep conditioner to nourish and hydrate your hair.

10. Style and maintain: Once your hair is dry, style it as desired. To maintain the color, use color-safe shampoos and conditioners, avoid

excessive heat styling, and protect your hair from UV rays.

Remember, these are general guidelines, and it's important to refer to the specific instructions provided by the hair color product you choose. Additionally, if you have any concerns or specific hair conditions, it's always recommended to consult a professional hairstylist for personalized advice and assistance.

Here are three more phrases related to coloring your hair:

1. How long should I leave the hair color on?

- The recommended development time varies depending on the hair color product. It's important to follow the instructions provided to achieve the best results.

2. Can I color my hair if it's already been chemically treated?

- It depends on the type of chemical treatment you've had. Some hair color products are designed to work on previously treated hair, while others may not be suitable. It's best to check the product instructions or consult a professional stylist for guidance.

3. How often should I touch up my roots?

- The frequency of root touch-ups depends on how quickly your hair grows and the contrast between your natural hair color and the dyed color. Typically, root touch-ups are done every 4-6 weeks, but it can vary for each individual.

Conversation example:

User: How long should I leave the hair color on?

Assistant: The recommended development time varies depending on the hair color product. It's important to follow the instructions provided to achieve the best results.

User: Can I color my hair if it's already been chemically treated?

Assistant: It depends on the type of chemical treatment you've had. Some hair color products are designed to work on previously treated hair, while others may not be suitable. It's best to check the product instructions or consult a professional stylist for guidance.

User: How often should I touch up my roots?

Assistant: The frequency of root touch-ups depends on how quickly your hair grows and the contrast between your natural hair color and the dyed color. Typically, root touch-ups are done every 4-6 weeks, but it can vary for each individual.

Natural, Organic, & Ammonia-Free Hair Dyes' Dirty Little Secret

The dirty little secret about natural, organic, and ammonia-free hair dyes is that while they may be marketed as healthier alternatives to conventional hair dyes, they still contain ingredients that can have potential risks and drawbacks.

1. Limited Color Options: Natural and organic hair dyes often have a more limited range of color options compared to conventional dyes. They may not be able to achieve certain vibrant or dramatic shades.

2. Less Long-Lasting Results: Ammonia-free and organic dyes tend to have shorter staying power and may fade more quickly compared to dyes that contain ammonia. This means you may need to touch up your hair more frequently to maintain the desired color.

3. Potential Allergic Reactions: Even though natural and organic dyes may use plant-based or herbal ingredients, they can still cause allergic reactions in some individuals. It's important to perform a patch test before applying the dye to your entire head to check for any adverse reactions.

4. Ineffective Gray Coverage: Natural and organic dyes may not provide as effective gray coverage as conventional dyes. They may require multiple applications or may not fully cover stubborn gray hairs.

5. Limited Lightening Power: If you're looking to lighten your hair or achieve a significant color change, natural and organic dyes may not be as effective as dyes containing ammonia or other chemical lightening agents.

6. Higher Cost: Natural and organic hair dyes are often more expensive than conventional dyes due to the use of higher quality ingredients and production methods.

It's important to note that "natural" and "organic" do not necessarily mean risk-free or without potential drawbacks. If you have specific concerns or sensitivities, it's best to consult with a professional hair colorist or dermatologist before using any hair dye product.

The Best Product To Cover Grays

There are several hair coloring products available that can effectively cover grays. The best product for covering grays can vary depending on individual preferences, hair type, and desired results. Here are some popular options:

1. Permanent Hair Color: Permanent hair color provides long-lasting results and complete coverage for gray hair. Look for a shade that closely matches your natural hair color or desired color.

2. Root Touch-Up Products: Root touch-up products are designed to specifically target and cover gray roots. They come in various forms such as sprays, powders, or creams and can provide temporary coverage until your next full coloring.

3. Demi-Permanent Hair Color: Demi-permanent hair color is a less harsh option that helps blend grays rather than fully covering them. It

provides a more natural and subtle result that gradually fades over time.

4. Henna Hair Dye: Henna is a natural plant-based dye that can cover grays while conditioning the hair. It is a more gentle and chemical-free option but may have limited color choices.

5. Hair Mascara or Temporary Color Sprays: These are quick and temporary solutions to cover grays. They provide temporary color that can be easily washed out. They are great for touch-ups or special occasions.

It's important to consider your hair type, color preferences, and any allergies or sensitivities before selecting a hair coloring product. It's also recommended to follow the instructions provided by the manufacturer and perform a patch test before applying the product to your entire hair. If you're unsure which product would be best for you, consulting a professional hairstylist can provide personalized recommendations.

Hairdressers Guide To Coloring Your Own Hair And Not Ruining It

Coloring your own hair can be a challenging task, but with proper guidance and precautions, you can achieve good results without ruining your hair. Here is a hairdresser's guide to coloring your own hair:

1. Choose the Right Color: Select a hair color that complements your skin tone and matches your desired result. Consider factors such as your natural hair color, the level of maintenance required, and any previous color treatments.

2. Read and Follow Instructions: Always thoroughly read the instructions provided with the hair color product. Follow the

recommended mixing ratios, processing times, and application techniques to ensure best results.

3. Perform a Strand Test: Before applying the color to your entire hair, perform a strand test. Take a small section of hair and apply the color according to the instructions. This will help you determine the processing time and how the color will turn out on your hair.

4. Prepare Your Hair: It's important to have clean and dry hair before coloring. Avoid applying any styling products or conditioner that may interfere with the color absorption. Protect your clothing and skin by wearing an old shirt and applying petroleum jelly or a barrier cream along your hairline and ears.

5. Apply the Color Properly: Section your hair into manageable parts and apply the color evenly from roots to ends. Use a brush or applicator provided with the hair color kit. Start with the roots and work your way down, ensuring every strand is covered. Comb through the hair to distribute the color evenly.

6. Time it Right: Follow the recommended processing time provided by the hair color product. Set a timer to avoid over-processing, which can damage your hair. If you're covering grays, you may need to leave the color on for a few extra minutes.

7. Rinse and Condition: Once the processing time is complete, rinse your hair thoroughly with lukewarm water until the water runs clear. Apply the conditioner provided in the kit or a deep conditioning treatment to restore moisture and smoothness to your hair.

8. Maintain Your Color: To prolong the life of your hair color, use color-safe shampoos and conditioners. Minimize exposure to direct sunlight, chlorinated water, and heat styling tools, as they can cause color fading.

9. Seek Professional Help: If you're unsure or have concerns about coloring your hair at home, it's recommended to consult a

professional hairdresser. They can provide personalized advice, recommend suitable products, and assist you in achieving your desired color.

Remember, coloring your own hair requires care and attention. If you're uncertain or have complex coloring needs, it's best to seek professional assistance to avoid potential damage or undesirable results.

Hairdresser Reacts To People Coloring Their Hair Using XMONDO Color

I can provide general information about XMONDO Color and how it is perceived by some hairdressers.

XMONDO Color is a hair color brand founded by Brad Mondo, a popular hairstylist and YouTuber. The brand offers a range of vibrant and fashion-forward hair color products, including semi-permanent and direct dye options. Many people are attracted to XMONDO Color due to its bold and unique shades, as well as its association with Brad Mondo's expertise in hair styling and color.

Hairdressers may have varying opinions about XMONDO Color and any other hair color brand. Some hairdressers appreciate the creativity and self-expression that XMONDO Color allows individuals to achieve with their hair. They may acknowledge the brand's popularity and the appeal of its vibrant shades among younger demographics.

However, it's worth noting that some professional hairdressers may have concerns or reservations about using non-professional or DIY hair color brands like XMONDO Color. These concerns can stem from factors such as the lack of professional supervision during application, the potential for improper color mixing or application techniques, and the risk of hair damage or undesirable results.

Hairdressers often emphasize the importance of proper hair care, color selection, and application techniques to achieve desired results while minimizing potential damage. They may recommend consulting with a professional stylist, especially for complex color transformations or if an individual has specific hair concerns or previous color treatments.

Ultimately, the reaction of a hairdresser to people using XMONDO Color or any other hair color brand will depend on their professional perspective, experience, and personal preferences. It's always a good idea to consult with a professional hairstylist for personalized advice and guidance when it comes to coloring your hair.

Specific Hair Types Or Conditions That Are Not Suitable For Coloring At Home

There are certain hair types or conditions that may not be suitable for coloring at home. Here are a few examples:

1. Damaged or Over-Processed Hair: If your hair is already damaged, weak, or over-processed from previous chemical treatments, it may not be in a healthy enough state to handle additional color processing. Coloring damaged hair can further weaken it and lead to breakage or excessive dryness. In such cases, it's best to consult with a professional hairdresser who can assess the condition of your hair and advise you on the best course of action.

2. Severe Hair or Scalp Conditions: If you have severe hair or scalp conditions such as open sores, infections, severe dandruff, or an irritated scalp, it is advisable to avoid coloring your hair at home. Chemical hair color products can irritate or worsen these conditions and may lead to discomfort or further damage. Seeking guidance from a dermatologist or hair care professional is recommended in such cases.

3. Uneven Hair Porosity: Hair porosity refers to how well your hair can absorb and retain moisture. If your hair has uneven porosity, meaning different parts of your hair absorb and hold color differently, achieving consistent and even results with at-home hair color products can be challenging. It may be best to consult with a professional stylist who can assess your hair's porosity and recommend the most suitable coloring techniques.

4. Dramatic Color Changes: If you're looking to make a drastic color change, especially from a significantly darker shade to a lighter one, it can be challenging to achieve the desired results at home. Lightening hair requires bleaching, a process that can be complex and potentially damaging if not done correctly. It's often best to consult with a professional colorist who has the expertise and experience to achieve the desired color safely and effectively.

Remember, every individual's hair is unique, and what may work for one person may not work for another. If you have any concerns or doubts about coloring your hair at home, it's always a good idea to consult with a professional hairdresser or colorist who can provide personalized advice based on your specific hair type, condition, and desired outcome.

Does Hair Coloring Wax Work

Hair coloring wax can work effectively for temporary hair color changes. Hair coloring wax is a type of hair product that contains pigments and wax-like ingredients. It is usually used to add temporary color highlights, streaks, or overall color to the hair without causing permanent damage or commitment.

Hair coloring wax is easy to apply and provides instant color results. It can be applied directly to dry hair, and the color can be built up by adding more product. Hair coloring wax is typically suitable for all hair types and colors.

However, it's important to note that hair coloring wax is temporary and can wash out easily with water or after a few shampoos. It is not as long-lasting as permanent or semi-permanent hair dyes. The color intensity and longevity may vary depending on factors such as hair porosity, the amount of product applied, and hair care routines.

Hair coloring wax is a popular choice for those who want to experiment with different hair colors temporarily, try out new looks for special occasions, or add vibrant accents to their hair without long-term commitment. It can be a fun and creative way to change your hair color temporarily.

If you're considering using hair coloring wax, it's recommended to do a patch test first to check for any adverse reactions or sensitivity. Additionally, follow the instructions provided by the specific product you choose for the best results.

As with any hair product, it's important to take proper care of your hair before and after using hair coloring wax. This includes keeping your hair well-moisturized, using a gentle shampoo and conditioner, and protecting your hair from excessive heat styling and UV exposure.

Overall, hair coloring wax can be a convenient and temporary solution for adding color to your hair, but it may not provide the same longevity and color options as permanent or semi-permanent hair dyes.

Can Hair Coloring Wax Be Used On All Hair Types, Or Is It More Suitable For Certain Textures

Hair coloring wax can generally be used on all hair types, including straight, wavy, curly, and coily hair. However, it's important to consider the specific characteristics of your hair when using hair coloring wax:

1. Lighter Hair Shades: Hair coloring wax tends to show up more vibrantly on lighter hair shades. If you have dark or very dark hair, the color may appear less intense or may not be as noticeable. In such cases, pre-lightening or bleaching the hair may be necessary to achieve the desired color result.

2. Porosity: Hair porosity refers to how well your hair can absorb and retain moisture. If you have highly porous hair, such as damaged or chemically treated hair, the color may be more easily absorbed and may appear more intense. On the other hand, low-porosity hair may be more resistant to absorbing the color, resulting in a less vibrant effect. It's important to consider your hair's porosity when using hair coloring wax.

3. Texture and Curl Pattern: Hair coloring wax can work on all hair textures, but the application and results may vary. On straight or wavy hair, the color may distribute more evenly and show up more prominently. However, on curly or coily hair, the color may appear less defined or may need more product and careful manipulation to ensure even coverage and color intensity.

4. Product Build-Up: Hair coloring wax can have a wax-like texture, which may create some build-up on the hair. This can be more noticeable on fine or thin hair types. It's important to use the product sparingly and wash your hair thoroughly to remove any residue after use.

It's always a good idea to do a patch test and strand test before using hair coloring wax on your entire head, especially if you have concerns about how it may interact with your specific hair type or condition. Additionally, following the instructions provided with the specific hair coloring wax product you choose will help ensure the best results for your hair.

Tips On How To Apply Hair Coloring Wax For The Best Results

Certainly! Here are some tips to help you achieve the best results when applying hair coloring wax:

1. Start with Clean and Dry Hair: Make sure your hair is clean and dry before applying hair coloring wax. This will help the wax adhere to the hair better and provide more even coverage.

2. Protect Your Clothing and Surfaces: Hair coloring wax can be messy, so it's a good idea to wear an old shirt or use a cape or towel to protect your clothing. Also, cover the surfaces around you with towels or plastic sheets to prevent any accidental staining.

3. Section Your Hair: To ensure even application, divide your hair into smaller sections using clips or hair ties. This will help you work through your hair systematically and avoid missing any areas.

4. Apply a Small Amount of Wax: Start with a small amount of hair coloring wax and rub it between your palms to warm it up. Then, apply it to the desired sections of your hair. Remember, a little goes a long way, so start with a modest amount and gradually add more if needed.

5. Work from Roots to Ends: Begin applying the wax at the roots of the hair and work your way down to the ends. This will help distribute the color evenly and create a natural-looking effect.

6. Use Fingers or Tools: You can apply the hair coloring wax using your fingers for a more casual and blended look. If you prefer more precise application, consider using a brush or sponge applicator designed for hair color.

7. Blend and Comb Through: After applying the wax, use your fingers or a wide-toothed comb to distribute the color and blend it into your hair. This will help create a seamless transition and avoid any harsh lines.

8. Style as Desired: Once you've achieved the desired color, you can style your hair as usual. Keep in mind that hair coloring wax can add texture and hold to your hair, so you may need to adjust your styling routine accordingly.

9. Seal the Color (Optional): If you want to enhance the longevity of the color, you can use a hair spray or setting spray to seal the hair coloring wax. This can help minimize transfer and extend the color's lifespan.

10. Layering Technique: If you want to achieve a more intense or vibrant color, you can apply multiple layers of hair coloring wax. After applying the first layer, wait for it to dry, and then add another layer on top until you reach the desired color intensity.

11. Experiment with Mixing Colors: Hair coloring wax is often available in a variety of shades. You can get creative and experiment by mixing different colors together to create your custom shade. This allows you to personalize your hair color and achieve unique results.

12. Use Heat for Better Absorption (Optional): Applying a small amount of heat, such as using a hairdryer on low heat, can help the hair coloring wax absorb better into the hair. This can enhance the color payoff and longevity. Be cautious not to apply excessive heat, as it can melt the wax or cause damage to the hair.

13. Set the Color with Powder (Optional): To increase the longevity of the hair coloring wax and reduce transfer, you can lightly dust your hair with a colorless setting powder. This can help set the wax and prevent it from rubbing off onto clothes or other surfaces.

14. Touch-Ups and Maintenance: Hair coloring wax is not a permanent solution, and the color will fade over time or with washing. To maintain the color, you may need to perform touch-ups as needed. Simply reapply the wax to the areas where the color has faded or become less vibrant.

15. Gentle Removal: When you're ready to remove the hair coloring wax, it can typically be washed out with regular shampoo. Make sure to thoroughly rinse your hair to remove any residue. You may need to shampoo your hair multiple times to ensure that all the wax is completely removed.

16. Hair Health and Maintenance: While hair coloring wax is temporary and generally less damaging than permanent dyes, it's still important to maintain the overall health of your hair. This includes following a regular hair care routine, using nourishing shampoos and conditioners, and avoiding excessive heat styling or other damaging practices.

Remember to follow the specific instructions provided with the hair coloring wax you're using, as different products may have slight variations in application techniques. Additionally, it's always a good idea to do a patch test and strand test before applying the wax to your entire head, especially if you're using a new product or have any concerns about potential reactions or color results.

How Does The Level And Tone Of Hair Color Affect The Final Result

The level and tone of hair color play a significant role in determining the final result of a hair color application. Here's how they affect the outcome:

1. Level: The level refers to the lightness or darkness of the hair color on a scale from 1 to 10, with 1 being the darkest (black) and 10 being the lightest (palest blonde). The level of the hair color you choose determines how much you'll need to lighten or darken your hair to achieve the desired result. For example, if you have dark brown hair (level 4) and want to achieve a light blonde shade (level 8), you'll need to lighten your hair by several levels.

2. Tone: The tone refers to the underlying hue or color present in the hair. It can be warm, cool, or neutral. Warm tones include red, orange, and yellow, while cool tones include blue, violet, and green. Neutral tones are balanced and not predominantly warm or cool. The tone you choose can significantly impact the overall look and feel of the hair color.

- Warm Tones: Warm-toned hair colors can add vibrancy and richness to the hair. They include shades like golden blonde, copper red, and caramel brown. Warm tones are often used to create a sun-kissed or natural-looking effect.

- Cool Tones: Cool-toned hair colors have undertones of blue, violet, or green. They can create ashy, platinum, or silver shades. Cool tones are commonly used to neutralize unwanted warmth in the hair or to achieve fashionable cool colors.

- Neutral Tones: Neutral-toned hair colors have a balanced mixture of warm and cool tones. They are often used to create natural-looking shades or to provide a more subtle color change.

When selecting a hair color, considering both the level and tone is essential to achieve the desired outcome. For example, choosing a level 6 (dark blonde) with a warm tone will result in a different appearance than choosing a level 6 with a cool or neutral tone.

It's important to consult with a professional stylist or refer to the specific color chart or swatches provided by the hair color brand you're using. Color charts typically display different shades at varying levels and tones, helping you visualize the potential outcome of your chosen hair color.

Additionally, factors such as the starting color of your hair, the condition of your hair, and any previous color treatments can also influence the final result. A professional stylist can assess these factors and help you make informed decisions to achieve your desired hair color outcome.

<u>Hair Color Theory 101 | Discover Kenra Color | Kenra Professional</u>

Hair Color Theory 101 is a term used to describe the basic principles and concepts behind hair color and the science behind it. It encompasses various aspects such as color wheel, color theory, hair color levels, undertones, and formulation techniques.

In Hair Color Theory 101, you will learn about the color wheel, which is a visual representation of colors arranged in a circular format. It helps in understanding color relationships and how different colors interact with each other. The color wheel is divided into primary colors (red, blue, and yellow), secondary colors (orange, green, and violet), and tertiary colors (a combination of primary and secondary colors).

Hair color levels refer to the darkness or lightness of the hair. It is measured on a scale from 1 to 10, with 1 being the darkest (black) and 10 being the lightest (pale blonde). Understanding hair color levels is essential for achieving the desired result when coloring hair.

Undertones are the underlying tones present in hair color. They can be warm (red, orange, yellow) or cool (blue, violet, green). Identifying the undertones in hair is crucial for selecting the right hair color shade and achieving desired results.

Formulation techniques involve the use of color formulas to achieve specific hair color results. This includes determining the amount of color to be used, the developer strength, and any additional additives or toners required.

Overall, Hair Color Theory 101 provides a foundation for understanding the principles of hair color and helps colorists or individuals interested in hair coloring to create beautiful and customized hair color results.

Example phrases with explanations:

1. Color wheel: The color wheel is a tool used in Hair Color Theory 101 to understand the relationships between different colors. It helps in selecting complementary or contrasting shades for hair color.

2. Levels and Tones: Hair color is often described in terms of levels and tones. The level refers to the lightness or darkness of the hair, with level 1 being the darkest black and level 10 being the lightest blonde. Tones refer to the underlying hues present in the hair, such as warm (red, orange, yellow) or cool (blue, violet, green) tones. Understanding hair color levels is important when choosing a hair color shade or determining the level of lift required for desired results.

3. Undertones: Undertones are the underlying tones present in hair color. Identifying the undertones in hair helps in selecting the right hair color shade and achieving accurate and flattering results.

4. Hair Pigments: Natural hair color is determined by the presence of pigments, primarily melanin. Melanin comes in two types: eumelanin, which ranges from dark brown to black, and pheomelanin, which ranges from yellow to red. The combination and concentration of these pigments determine the natural hair color.

5. Color Depth: Color depth refers to the intensity or saturation of a hair color. It can range from a soft, subtle hue to a bold, vibrant shade. Depth is achieved by adding or removing pigments to alter the intensity of the color.

6. Warm and Cool Colors: Understanding warm and cool colors is essential in formulating hair color. Warm colors, such as reds and oranges, add warmth and vibrancy to the hair. Cool colors, such as blues and violets, neutralize unwanted warm tones and create cooler, ashier shades.

7. Color Correction: In hair color correction, the principles of color theory are used to correct and balance unwanted tones or achieve desired results. For example, if hair has unwanted brassy or orange tones, a colorist may use a cool-toned color to neutralize the warmth.

8. Developer or Peroxide: Developer, also known as peroxide, is an essential component in hair color formulations. It helps to activate the color molecules and lift or deposit the color onto the hair. Different levels of developers, such as 10-volume, 20-volume, or 30-volume, provide varying degrees of lift and color deposit.

Short conversation example:

Person A: "I'm learning about Hair Color Theory 101. Can you explain what the color wheel is?"

Person B: "Sure! In Hair Color Theory 101, the color wheel is a visual representation of colors arranged in a circular format. It helps us understand the relationships between different colors and select complementary or contrasting shades for hair color."

Person A: "That makes sense! So, the color wheel helps us choose which colors to use for hair coloring?"

Person B: "Exactly! By using the color wheel, we can determine which colors will work well together and create the desired hair color result."